About Dean Fraser

Love is quite simply the most powerful creative force, self-healing energy and gift to wellbeing that exists. This book is dedicated to all us seekers of more than a treadmill existence - those looking to have a fuller, happier experience on this amazing planet of ours! - DEAN FRASER

Dean Fraser shows how evolving comes from living, making mistakes which are not really mistakes but learning, walking our talk and sometimes tripping up a few times before we finally get the message about what we need in order to grow - NEW DAWN MAGAZINE

KARMA IS QUANTUM ENERGY

Dean Fraser

Love is quite simply the most powerful creative force, self-healing energy and gift to wellbeing that exists...

Dean Fraser

CONTENTS

THIS BOOK HONOURS YOU!

Introduction - Karma Is Quantum Energy

Could it be that there is some arbitrary force at work, controlling what happens in our lives? This hidden, mysterious power that ensures we must pass through certain experiences in order to grow as people?

Certainly this is often how karma is perceived in popular culture. Patterns that just sort of... happen...probably for us to grow, we are just not quite sure exactly how.

When I look back through my own life, there were clearly obvious patterns, ways of reacting in different situations that, for a while at least, had become ingrained and pretty standard responses I rolled out whenever certain situations triggered them.

Often these emotional reactions can cause us to feel fundamentally uncomfortable within ourselves. Signs from our Higher Selves it is now time to react in a different way, the current paradigm no longer working.

Karma is in reality remarkably simple. Karma is simply our built-up emotional responses to different emotional triggers.

These triggers can manifest in many ways.

Through a confrontational situation, a piece of music, the changing seasons of the year, the smell of cooking, certain colours, photographs; in fact just about anything no matter how random it may appear to be can trigger an emotional response which makes us feel uncomfortable.

Now these responses could be as a result of experiences we have gone through in the current timeline of our life. They could be passed on through our DNA from our parents or ancestors, race memory or even from unresolved issues carried over from previous incarnations (a subject for another book I will write).

For the journey together we are taking I will focus solely on our own direct experiences in this life and the reality we create around us.

I should also add at this point, some emotional triggers can also make us feel warm inside and generally fantastic, these are indications of a nice balance and harmony surrounding those particular feelings.

Karma is not some mysterious Universal force at work that obliges us to go through certain hardships and then we can become a better person. The reality is that Karma is totally within our own control. We are the force responsible for our own karmic destiny. Our karmic taskmaster is us! Who could genuinely know what is best for us, other than ourselves?

So we are the ones in the driving seat when it comes to karma…

What I aim to give you are the keys to unlock your own future through healing the past.

Can you change your karma?

Most definitely YES!

Karma can also often be holding on to those repressed un-expressed feelings from even quite early childhood. Times we really wanted to express how we felt and were told to be quiet or when we came to realise that in order to be socially accepted we needed to supress a certain part of ourselves. Then when a situation occurs that triggers a similar response in ourselves to whatever feeling we repressed way-back-when, it results in often surprising levels of supressed anger manifesting, depression and feelings of life being unfair.

As a child I loved art. Quite early in life I discovered Surrealism through picture books showing the works of Salvador Dali and Rene Magritte. Naturally this influenced my childhood art; and to my delight at nine years' old I found some of my paintings exhibited in a local art exhibition. Even more delightedly I received certificates of commendation from the judges.

In secondary school, however, I came across an art teacher who strongly disliked Surrealism. Highly negatively critical of my art, she insisted I paint in Realism instead, which I obviously felt unhappy at the prospect of.

When faced with a still-life vase of flowers she would tell me quite loudly in front of all the class how my painting looked absolutely nothing like that vase of flowers! I tried in vain explaining how I had painted the flowers the way I interpreted them, but it fell upon deaf ears.

The long-term consequence of this childhood experience saw me falling out of love with art for many years and getting triggered to feel quite angry whenever accidentally encountering still-life realist paintings. My reaction to this teacher's words influenced my adult life all the way through into my mid-30's.

Eventually, with the encouragement of my significant other, I started visiting some Surrealist Art Galleries; and finally acquired some coloured pencils and a sketch-pad. Art is now once more a central part of my life...and I am still a Surrealist.

Any reaction we feel in any situation which is damaging us in some way is nearly always because of those unresolved emotions that were never allowed to be expressed back in childhood. Unresolved emotions cause blockages stopping us from truly feeling. Failing to allow us to be our Authentic Self.

These reactions manifest in many ways, through feelings of futility or frustration with the way our life functions.

Another unfortunate by product of any emotional blockages, if left undealt with, is they can create mental health issues and ultimately actual physical illnesses.

If we find ourselves reacting in certain set ways when the similar situations occur, and these emotional trigger responses make us feel uncomfortable or seem illogical, particularly to ourselves, then we are experiencing karma in action.

Overcoming karma is to overcome our own set way of looking at firstly ourselves and then the outer world, our interactions with everything and everyone in our life based on our built-up experiences.

All situations that occur in which we react by our own set of well-established rules, yet which seems to somehow take us further away from our objectives or makes it more difficult for others to see our point of view, are based on some long distant occurrence in our past; in other words engrained emotional responses.

These reactions often come across as totally irrational to others and perhaps more importantly even to ourselves!

I will share another example of this from my own life. A story I did allude to briefly once before in another book, but I sense is worth sharing this time in more detail for the truths it illustrates. How one small incident from childhood can continue to influence us throughout adult life and it is only when we are able to meditate upon it then the root cause can become apparent.

By the way, by meditation I am not necessarily talking about transcendental meditation here, although this is a wonderful way of calming the mind, what I mean is spending some time pondering a triggered feeling in depth and WHY these situations makes us feel a certain way. Turning inwards intuitively to know more about the truth of what is behind that feeling.

My example is one that started to become more obvious from my late teens into mature adulthood. I possessed an absolute fear of large ships and the thought of being on the water in one, especially deep water, would terrify me.

I am talking here about how even seeing a picture of a large ship would make me feel uncomfortable and my heart race a little faster.

Naturally, there then came a point where a journey on a large trans-channel ferry became inevitable. What we fear the most we do attract towards us, how else if we are going to be able to deal with it and move on?

The ferry journey was sprung upon me the day of travelling, I had no time to think too much about it or build up my deep-rooted fear reaction. I lived in Kent at that time, so it was just a short journey to Dover and then the ferry ride to Calais. I spent the whole journey across the English Channel, there locked in the gents, being really rather not terribly well…

Once I crawled off the ferry in Calais I began to think. I had actually done it, been on that ferry and survived! And yet the sense of fear at the prospect of the return journey was almost overwhelming me. I believe I would have rather swum back across the Channel!!!

Fate took a hand in events, okay I now know it was my higher-self working with me, however, at the time I thought it was fate. Rough seas meant that the return ferry had been cancelled and we found ourselves staying the night in Calais.

I began to think as I sat there watching the rough sea on that cold winter's evening, where my fear of ships and the deep sea had all originated from. I went back through my own timeline, pondering different events in my life.

Nobody I knew directly had ever died at sea, and no accidents involving ships in my family history. I thought about when I first became aware of the reality of big ships in any kind of tangible way.

Then as I journeyed back I remembered being a five-year-old in year one at school and finding a children's history book in the library. It was all about the Titanic and as a child with a very vivid imagination, when I read a book I imagined myself being right there in the horrific adventure taking place within the pages. This Titanic book had scared the living daylights out of me as I imagined this giant ship sinking to the bottom of the sea and me there in the cold, icy water.

One half hour read when I was five years old had gone on to affect my entire adult life. I laughed with relief when I realised that all the anxiety I had been suffering with for all those years and the limitations I had caused myself had all originated from my well-developed imagination and a children's picture book!

Needless to say the return journey to Dover the following morning was much more comfortable which I spent it out on deck watching the waves hitting the bow of the ship. And I have since happily been on boats of all sizes without any feelings of panic.

This is exactly what we can all do. Phobias, fears and misplaced anger will all have their root in some perhaps long consciously forgotten incident that happened or we witnessed.

If you have a phobia, think about when you first really felt it. Where in your personal history did you become aware of this reaction? If you have a fear of spiders, for example, as a small child did you witness someone else reacting in fear at the sight of a spider? If you have a fear of flying, perhaps you read something or saw an incident on television that featured a plane crash or a documentary that questioned the safety of flying?

I could go on giving examples, anyway nearly always phobias will have their roots in some often long forgotten occurrence in our own past.

Or they are passed on from our parents and if we do come to this realization, that we have been walking around limiting ourselves because of an inherited pattern of behaviour, then we can take action to do something about it and heal ourselves. We will go through how shortly.

If you have a poor relationship with money what were your experiences growing up? How did your parents or guardians explain to you when you wanted something in a shop that you could not have it? If it was in terms of "we cannot afford that" or "there isn't enough money to buy you things all the time" then it could well have set up feelings of anxiety around money, that there is never enough for everything and that will then be the vibration that is sent out there into quantum soup, creating a self-fulfilling prophecy.

The tools are right there within all of us to overcome any of our self-imposed limitations to become free of anxiety and panic responses to situations.

Then there is the other anxiety that is created by our own actions in the past and if they harmed another, the guilt that is carried around deep inside relating to that action.

Guilt and feelings of negativity about ourselves are also karma; or more specifically they create blockages in the good flow of energy or chi within and without us. Stopping us from realising our potential. Living authentically.

Guilt about an action we perpetrated can eat us up inside. even if we do not consciously give it much or any thought. Our cells will still nevertheless contain a memory of the event and we subconsciously do still feel it. The cells of our bodies store the memory of everything that happens in our life. On a quantum level our past literally creates exactly who we are...spiritually and physically.

Guilt carried around sends out the energy into the Universe that we are somehow unworthy of good things happening to us. And the Universe, as always, says "ok, lets' make it so". Sadly leading to experiencing a life of limitation. Then because of lack of self-worth, to the likelihood of more actions of negativity and the subsequent feelings of guilt that will lead to more lack of self-worth...and so it goes on and on and on...

Patterns of behaviour, and by this I mean both ones that lead to negative or positive feelings about ourselves creating energy that surrounds us, we then project out there into the Universe, creating our reality, every second, of every minute, of every single day of our lives.

There can be no escaping from this universal truth. Until we decide to create a new paradigm for ourselves, to build the kind of future we actually want, our personal energy projections will keep on giving us pretty much what we always had.

The other point we need to consider here is that if our cells contain the memory of all our actions, others who are more receptive will be able to actually feel this energy coming from us.

Have you ever met a person for the first time and shaken hands and immediately been attracted or repulsed by what you felt when you touched them? Congratulations, you are tuned into the energies of the Universe at a cellular level!

When you touched this new person, you picked up on their own cell memory. This kind of reaction is something people feel all the time and yet most of them tend to ignore it or find some reason to explain away the feeling. It is cellular communication and my intuition tells me that as this century progresses that this will become more the accepted normality as it is more understood.

Creating Our Own Future

The concept of balancing karma has become part of popular culture. There are thousands of books written on the subject and many people treat karma as an absolute reality. Balancing karma today is in essence still exactly the same as the great wisdoms of the ancients who talked about karma. In modern times though we tend to describe it in terms of the psychology of dealing with unresolved issues to then move on into a freedom from limitation.

Our psychological make up can obviously dramatically affect our physical and mental well-being. I have experienced how the power of thoughts and words directly influences the health of individuals myself and those I have helped throughout my several decades of experience. Sometimes in an incredibly positive way.

Suppressed emotions and/or misplaced reactions cause us stress.

It seems almost too obvious to state that if we are stressed and full of anxiety we are hardly likely to be functioning to the best of our ability. It goes further than that though. It is unresolved emotional issues, from whatever source, that will often have caused that stress. And this then permeates through our cells.

Surely then what is needed is a way to let go of reactions and such self-defeating behaviour patterns...

The good news is that most assuredly there is a way. A way to deal with the past experiences we are still carrying forward every single day or to put it another way, our karma.

The challenge is that it can take dedicated effort and the sincere desire to live a more auspicious life. Much travelling back through our own timeline will be needed, to more than likely traumatic experiences.

Although having said that, it is not always those traumatic experiences that shape us and make us who we are. There are cases where too much kindness can in fact be as harmful to growth and living life to the full as any negative experiences can be. The child growing up having every possible material whim satisfied is also going to have some adjusting to do as an adult going out into the big wide World once they realise that they will have to create their own future and life.

Pondering deeply about how the feelings that events that occurred in our past created in us and how they are carried forward is simply the way to freedom. What emotional responses manifest when we meditate upon past disharmony?

Or focussing on hurts we may have inflicted on others and how we felt at the time. What made us react in that particular way? Is it through something that occurred in our own timeline, a conditioned response that when the same event presented itself we went down that same personal road most travelled?

Sometimes these are such small incidents as to have been long lost to conscious memory, however, the emotional response we feel to a certain experience will still trigger a latent memory and so we react.

In the case of myself there were countless examples of such incidents and issues, I have dealt with many and yet I am still discovering some of them now. I spent many nights as I went to sleep pondering different points in my life and pivotal moments that occurred, and then as I drifted into my dreams I asked for the answers the following day to be shown.

And for sure they always were, often in the most bizarre way...like seeing a van drive past with a certain slogan on the side that related to exactly what I had been focussing on or something I overheard a stranger saying on their phone as they walked by; and then comes the eureka moment and enlightenment!

I am sure you will have similar experiences should you decide that it is time to walk the path to personal freedom and free will. You too will experience the amazement and excitement when some answer to a question is given in a most abstract and bizarre way. It becomes second nature after a while to absolutely expect to gain wisdoms about our karma and it is what we do with these wisdoms, that of course, shape our future destiny.

If there are any issues you know it is long overdue for you to deal with ponder them as you fall asleep and expect to gain greater understanding soon. And know it will happen for you.

Let's get practical next...and begin the pathway to a new paradigm...

Walking Our Talk Through Love

The primary way to cleanse ourselves of self-limiting thought patterns and unpleasant irrational reactions is simply this.

Forgiveness.

Sounds simple doesn't it?

In essence it is. Forgiveness.

In practice though it can take us on a long journey back through our life and frequently a challenging one at that. To seemingly tiny events that shaped who we are and what our lives have become.

To balance karma is to forgive those who we feel have wronged us in some way. And also, importantly forgive ourselves for mistakes we feel that we may have made, those we sense have brought us to where we are in life.

Forgiveness is absolutely the best thing we can do for ourself. And this includes forgiving ourselves for any hurts we may have perpetrated upon others.

And by forgive I mean to let go in every possible sense of the anger and any feeling of injustice, any guilt, that the original incident caused us to experience.

We have to absolutely feel the time and place the event occurred as if we are there now and focus deeply on our emotions. It may take more than one visit to the event to be able to get to the stage of feeling forgiveness. All kinds of trauma can be brought to the surface. We need to give ourselves time to deal with the latent buried issues that are now there to be addressed. There isn't a clock ticking here, however long the healing takes is fine.

It is the ultimate peace of mind and closure we achieve which matters.

Regardless of the situation or people involved the important thing is to get to the point where it is possible to forgive. By this I mean genuinely forgive from within. Sending love into the situation and healing it.

Love is the soothing balm that heals the past.

It bears repeating that forgiving ourselves and others is actually the single greatest favour we can do for ourselves. Forgiveness and feeling love instead frees us from having to go through the same emotional responses continually, like for example the next time when a similar situation occurs.

This time the event will be looked at in a completely different way, with gratitude. Closure having now been made and more freedom gained.

I should make it clear that feeling forgiveness is a very personal process, if someone in your past has done you serious harm and you have lived with that all your life, still feeling the anger and injustice...then I am compassionately sorry to have to tell you that sadly the situation is still controlling you. Reach deep down inside and see if there is any light there? If there is a possible way to lay the trauma to rest and feel differently about the situation. Much peace and love I send to you on your journey to healing.

I am asked about forgiveness and if it is necessary to tell the person, if that is possible, that we have forgiven them for some occurrence long ago. Or indeed to ask forgiveness from a person we have hurt.

The simple answer to this is no it is not.

Forgiveness is about ourselves and how we feel, the emotional healing that comes from bringing love into a previously unresolved event in our own past is all. There is absolutely no need at all for the person or persons involved in the event to know that you have gone through the process of forgiving them through love.

Strangely enough though, as the vibration surrounding the event has now changed and the emotions we feel are now calm, it quite often happens that the person or persons involved, if they are able to, will also respond to you in a different way than before.

On a cellular level you will feel different to them, that combined with the changed energy you are sending out can make them react quite dramatically differently to you. And even if they don't, at least you now know that it is only because their karma is not yet resolved and they are still a way off from escaping the quantum see-saw of cause and effect.

We talked earlier about the power of our thoughts and minds to create our reality. This is what forgiveness is really all about.

Sending out the right signals through firstly our thoughts, which are powerful energy vibrations our feelings about whatever we are dealing with and then our words.

Words carry those emotions we are feeling at any given time giving power to our thoughts. So what we clearly desire then is for these feelings, and words to be in harmony and filled with love. To sincerely no longer subconsciously wish harm to others, those who we previously had issues with. After a while it becomes second nature to develop a positive minded approach to life, one which ensures we never create more negative karma through our actions.

Then we can be said to be in balanced karma. For sure, there will still be challenging times to face, however, if we are balanced and centred within ourselves then we are better equipped to deal with them. We can go through these challenges staying true to our essence and who we are.

Everybody Goofs-Up Sometimes

We have all done it. Made those decisions that if we could only go back and change things, we might have done things differently, said something different or maybe not even said anything at all!

We need to ensure these goofing-up moments never define who we are now. Yes, for sure, on that one occasion we did not necessarily do things with the best of intentions, perhaps for ourselves or even others. Or else we just downright made a mistake!

Mistakes are only learning how to not do things.

Even Holistic Lifestyle Coaches goof-up!

Failing to back-up the files for this very book led to me losing nearly a year's worth of manuscript after my computer crashed to the point of oblivion. Starting from scratch again ended up my only choice. Which I actually ended up doing nearly seven years later, strangely enough...

I believe events happen for reasons. Losing my original files made me realise I needed more experience before making public this particular book. Whilst I cannot say I was delighted to lose all that original work; with the benefit of hindsight I can see precisely why it happened.

We have all experienced goofing-up...mistakes or failures never, ever define who we are. EVER! But they can make us wiser.

A Final Word About Forgiveness

As we discussed earlier, love is the soothing balm that heals the past.

I cannot overstate that forgiving ourselves and others is actually the single greatest favour we can do for ourselves. Forgiveness and feeling love completely frees us from having to go through the same traumatic emotional responses continually.

The next occasion a similar situation occurs we are free!

This time the event will be looked at in a completely different way. With gratitude for the self-healing that has now taken place. Closure has been made.

We all walk our own path towards becoming the ultimate version of our own multi-dimensional being, represented here on Earth in our human form. As we are all in fact multi-dimensional beings travelling around during our waking hours in human form, surely it must make perfect sense then to nurture and look after ourselves in the best way possible? Yes?

It is essential to love ourselves.

How we will develop into the ultimate happy and enthusiastic person is through love. And this is all part of the process to accepting ourselves. Perceived faults as well!

Maybe you want to lead a more auspicious life and yet still struggle to come to terms with some part of yourself you have trouble accepting?

If there is some aspect of your personality or reactions in certain situations that is troubling you have every reason to be feeling deeply happy. That you are even aware enough to actually be concerned and also if something feels so wrong it can surely be changed.

A polarity exists within all of us. Call it yin and yang, positive and negative or light and dark. Whatever label we place upon it, part of living in a human body is to know this polarity. Bring to mind people you know; it is certainly easy to see examples of both extremes of this polarity in action.

The wonderful thing about the people we meet is our reaction to them, how they make us feel. The person who comes across as overly critical or judgemental is far from being at ease within themselves. Those who point fingers at others and ridicule are struggling with some part of who they are, something that makes them feel uncomfortable and ill at ease about their own inner self. Transversely those who are comfortable in their own skin and at peace within will very rarely behave in an overly critical way or be unpleasantly judgemental. A person's behaviour says a lot about how they feel about themselves.

We need to come to the point of acceptance. Our own faults are showing us something about ourselves and these can be worked on. We need to embrace them and come to appreciate them. If we find that there is some part of our basic personality or our emotional reactions in certain situations that is troubling to us, we have the tools within us to transform and let them go.

We need to send our own loving energy into our own perceived faults. Alter the emotions which surround them. Transformational change can then begin.

Questioning is the beginning of wisdom. And questioning our own nature shows a desire to know ourselves better, this is the deepest wisdom.

We need to forgive ourselves through love for any hurts our own actions may have caused and trace back where that pattern of behaviour originated from in order for it to also be healed through love. Only then can we move a little further towards complete freedom.

Self-Love Is Vitally Important

Without self-love how are we to share our love with others?

How to get to the point of self-love?

Well, by firstly finding just one part of yourself that you are happy with. Something about you which works well for you and always makes you feel happy. An aspect of who you are that sits so well with you that you would never wish to change in any way. In order to plant the smallest acorn of self-love in the subconscious, focus on and really ponder how this wonderful part of you makes you feel when you think about it. Enjoy the warmth of the emotion.

First step now taken; we are well on our way! Let us see how to bring that feeling into other parts of life and begin to transform, in order to feel this fabulous across the whole spectrum of you.

We will usually have something within the vast range of emotions, feelings and reactions which we will wish to work upon to subsequently become more at peace within ourselves.

Again, ponder deeply the nice feelings associated with the "good" part of you. And now move your thoughts to think about some other aspect of you that you sense needs some work. This can be anything you dislike in your reactions or patterns of thinking.

It is important here to only concentrate on the one aspect at once. As you think about how this challenging part of you makes you feel, start to remember those beautiful warm feelings you experienced a few moments ago. Feel them! Really feel them!!!

It is going to take practise to master this exercise. I can promise you this though, the more often you undertake setting aside time in order to concentrate on this, the more results you will get. What is happening here is the start of a transformational process, a self-healing to welcome self-love into your life. Re-programming issues and healing them. And more importantly feeling far more comfortable in your own skin and within who you are.

As each issue is transformed the easier it gets and you will begin to experience the sense of a different approach to life starting to happen for you.

What Do You Want?

Deciding what it is you really want from life...

Okay I'm thinking you are probably wondering what the heck I'm talking about, yes? Surely all of us want to be happy and successful, don't we?

Well that all depends. You would be amazed how baggage from the past can block us from achieving all we could. We need to fundamentally feel WORTHY of achieving happiness and success.

And we also need to be aware that actual success can take many forms as well as only achieving material wealth. It needs to encompass all the areas of our lives such as health goals ticked-off as achieved or feeling truly at one and peace within who we are...

If you find it challenging to buy into feeling worthy of success then acquire a positivity self-hypnosis CD from your bookstore/library or download something from a source intuition tells you that you can trust on the internet.

And take some time forgiving those in your past such as parents or teachers for those times when they unintentionally programmed you with limitations in mindset. Clearly they usually never mean to do this they are just running their own internal programs through life and once you are living your ideal reality you can be an example to all of your family and friends about just what it is possible to achieve from this life.

Let's get back to this "what do you really want?" question. As we established this is all down to what success means to you. To some this is likely be limitless amounts of cash, to others the freedom to do what they want without having to budget too much.

Personally speaking, my definition of success was initially all about living stress-free and actually allowing myself to relax enough to genuinely enjoy life!

Take some time to do this, think deeply about what you really want and that is half the trick complete...more about this later. For now...

What Do You Never Want?

Well, for sure there is one proven way to attract to us the things we don't want and that is to constantly think about not wanting them. And tell everyone around us how much we don't want them. The energy of our thoughts works the same way always.

What we think about all the time, what we focus on, what we talk about – all becomes our reality, and this includes all those things we don't want to happen, which we put so much energy into not wanting.

So, if you and I are spending all our time focussing on and talking about stress, depression or feeling unwell, then we cannot feel too shocked when those things will be the reality of our day-to-day life...

Indecision Sends Out A Powerful Message Of Limitation

As we have now established what we think about constantly creates our reality, in every single sense, every single time without cessation.

And this works equally well with the things we fear, just as strongly as it does with those more positive experiences we would rather attract into our lives.

Yet, there is an upside here! The rather cool reality about all those negative thoughts is that if we wish for something to not happen, it does take infinitely more effort than wishing for some good positive outcome instead. And does take far longer to manifest that negative thought in our lives as well.

For sure constant vigilance is needed, there is some good news though.

The upside is that clearly here it has to be entirely possible to completely change our lives by simply changing our minds, what we focus on.

Thinking about what we DO want, keeping our focus positively and fixed on those results we actually desire to happen.

Keep our thoughts good and positive and life will always be interesting, for sure there will still be challenges (it's how we grow as people!), however, with a more positive attitude within our feelings and the power of words or how we choose to verbally express ourselves (which is vitally important), we can enjoy a massively more harmonious life.

Expectation does create the life that we live.

Believe It Can Happen

If you and I ever really want to achieve anything new and amazing, then we need to believe it firstly unequivocally is possible for it to happen! It needs to become as natural as opening your front door, you put that key in the lock and you are home.

Belief is the unwavering inner knowing that what we desire can genuinely surely happen. We might not yet know exactly how it is all going to play out, although in truth the physical details are actually unimportant. The important part is the belief that it can happen and preparedness to take personal action once the moment arrives to show itself, as it surely will.

Taking Action

Nothing interesting ever happens in the life of sedentary people.

For us though, first comes the expectation of results and secondly some clear action which needs to be taken to be able to bring about whatever we desire.

After the genuine expectation (Energy), then later comes our part of the deal to fulfil and virtually every single time this is going to require the leaving of comfort zones and getting directly personally involved with the ultimate outcome.

Once you have been working for a while with consciously projecting your Energy it becomes second nature to become aware of the time arriving for action when it makes its presence known. This is the moment to truly come alive and invest those actions with a nice healthy dose of enthusiasm and passion. Together with the thanks and gratitude you will naturally feel for another dream becoming the reality of your life.

The man who once had a vision to revolutionize production line technology, Henry Ford once said something along the lines of "If you think you can or cannot do a thing, you're absolutely right".

Integrity

Being a person of our word is vitally important. When making promises ensuring we can fulfil the commitment we made. If for some unforeseen reason circumstances change and render following through on a promise impossible, explaining how and why to whoever it affects in ample time before the allotted moment of fulfilment. And if possible then following through at the soonest opportunity later.

It goes without saying if we wish to be taken seriously, considered trustworthy and respected, we need to behave with impeccable integrity. Keeping those words we say together with our actions, honest and open to scrutiny by anyone.

Having made the decision to live your life with integrity, you must be honest with yourself first and foremost. Have there ever been any occasions relating to your past behaviour where perhaps you have sailed a little close to the wind, been economical with the truth for personal gain or to avoid the consequences of your actions?

If this is the case, that's awesome, the fact you are honest enough with yourself to accept this is brilliant. And what next, is it time to move on and leave it all behind you now? Well, almost...

If you have this kind of past, then know for sure that you are going to be tested. Do you genuinely possess the kind of integrity you are projecting now or is it just skin deep? Situations occurring in your life allowing you to show your true mettle and your resistance to the temptation of falling back into those old comfort zones.

Being a person of integrity may not always win you thousands of friends, it is certainly going to attract the right one's though!

Looking Laterally

I took a sabbatical for a year as I wrote the original transcript of this book and reclusively did not commit to any live coaching events or promote myself as open for business. The question when returning to the arena of my usual work became how to quickly re-establish myself. The business world changes incredibly quickly and taking myself out of the game for a year inevitably I found myself also out of the loop commercially.

Without planning it all out too much I did have an intuitive sense of how to not only now get myself once more out in front of people, I had the feeling I might actually be able to do this in a way where my profile would be raised far beyond anything I had ever considered possible before...

This time round I knew I wanted to reach out to help people all around the world.

Firstly, I set up my events, publishing and admin company Alive To Thrive Ltd to handle the day to day running of my diary ensuring I honoured all of my commitments.

Next I used all of my three decades plus of communication experience to get commissions writing self-help articles for numerous magazines absolutely right across the globe, while enjoying the by-product of the outrageous level of publicity this naturally generated!

I gave interviews in whatever media, whenever they were requested; and also sent paper and digital copies of my other books all over the world to be reviewed.

Giving myself the target of reaching at least five new contacts every single day and by working diligently for over a year, I got there. I became an "overnight" success story through trusting my message would step-up to work on a global scale. I happily found my opinion also now sought out at a spectacularly higher level than I ever enjoyed prior to my writing year out.

Each year since I can easily reach in excess of ten million people through my books, audios, live shows, radio and above all my columns for magazines. Had I not taken that year out I am convinced I would never have seen the bigger picture and enthusiastically gone for this global presence. And yet this option was there all the time, hiding in plain sight.

What skills do you already have? Are you in possession of something which perhaps only requires a little lateral thought and the right marketing to give you everything you might wish for?

Making It Last

If we love the thought of wearing a designer suit each day, but our success mindset is incongruent with this reality, we will never feel at ease within that lifestyle. It will feel odd or like we are playing dress-up!

Re-read this book until you feel able to let-go of anything at all which might hold you back within your thoughts or mindsets. Living rich is never only about our bank balance, it is crucially feeling comfortable within success and whatever that personally means to us.

Butterfly Minds

So, there we are putting out all that fantastic energy and yet the changes we have initiated seem to develop so far...then...slowly...stop.

Often we seem to have this immense difficulty in deciding what we really want from life and change our minds every other week about:

1. What kind of career we would like.

2. Where we wish to live and in what kind of house.

3. What success really means to us.

4. Which car to drive.

5. If we wish to be single or married.

6. What kind of further education to enrol for.

7. Or even what kind of parties we will host once we are successful!

You get the picture, keep changing our mind and all our personal energy is dissipated.

To go through building our focussed energy up all over again as we home-in instead on the latest version of the new successful life we wish to live...until the next time we change our minds...and then it all needs to start over once more!

Spend plenty of seriously fun time mapping out what you genuinely want your life to look like.

Rather than metaphorically deciding you want a beach house and then a week later realising a penthouse apartment is more you so you will have that instead...and then the next week perhaps after all you will just live on your yacht-with-a-view; we need to do our best to stick to our dreams!

That is why it is vitally important, before even beginning on the path to personal freedom, to at least have some vision of where you are actually heading...

Those routes to getting there evolve as we travel towards dreams, which is a different matter altogether and as we will see throughout our journey together this is truly an essential and exciting part of the process.

In the meantime, it is extremely useful to keep at the forefront of your mind when thinking about the future you are shaping for yourself - this or something even better!

Then if the personal concept of your own success is any way inadvertently limiting all that you might TRULY achieve – you are instead allowing your even potentially higher achievements the opportunity to really happen!

Controlled Power

If you lose control of yourself, you lose control of the situation and your ability to be empowered. Anger and frustration take away your personal power...always.

Spiritually Successful

We have all have more than likely met a few of those single-minded spiritually focussed people. They all share one thing in common. They devote themselves solely to personal development with the utmost zeal and are like sponges soaking up ways to spiritually grow. The other personality trait they often unfortunately share (and express this often) is how they certainly do not need money and in fact dislike having possessions. You guessed it, they are all struggling financially to get by.

Often some people seem to be under the illusion that spirituality and success are somehow separate entities. Maybe we can have one or the other, but definitely not both. This is patently untrue, for absolute proof of this take the time to read a few autobiographies of those hugely successful ethical businesspeople, martial arts legends and global adventurers.

You all know the ones, those individuals who became materially successful without every sacrificing the core essence of their ethics, who they are within themselves and how they choose to treat others.

It has even been suggested by some that focusing on making money might be the root of all evil.

Wow!

Talk about setting up a self-defeating negative vision of success!

Surely possessive greed and failing to use wealth to help others is way more negatively-minded than ethically working for the money you deserve by Universal Law to enter your life?

Money has energy which is neither positive nor negative of itself. It is what WE choose to do that determines the frequency of our wealth energy wave and frankly more importantly if our success makes us feel happy and healthy.

Money doesn't care if we are devoutly religious, on our own personal path to spiritual enlightenment or at the other end of the scale eschew spirituality all together.

We all have the freedom of choice to grow into our dreams and if that includes being wealthy, then we all begin from the same starting place regardless of background. It is all about mindset and listening to our intuition to let it guide us into direct action when required. Changing the energy of our lives always requires we first act to transform things within our mindset of what is possible.

The sponge analogy I used before is good, let us adopt that. How about we become sponges to soak up anything which can help us grow as individuals? Whatever that personally means to you or me.

If that turn out to be financially, spiritually and ideally both simultaneously, then we are living about perfectly!

Words Can Do So Much

As our thoughts create energy, then the words we choose to use are the force that helps our reality to manifest.

Have you ever noticed those individuals who constantly use expletives and express themselves in an unusually harsh way, very rarely seem to be exactly happy people? I am sure you will all know of at least one person who falls into that category.

Think of people in the public eye as well. Those who seem aggressive and angry, using extreme ways of expressing themselves, very rarely come across as spectacular shining examples of how to get life right and be happy forever.

Thoughts + words = reality...ours.

These are so many examples of potential greatness stifled by the choice of using limiting thoughts and words. And it really is a choice. We are the ones in charge of what we choose to primarily think about and the words we choose to express ourselves with.

Is It Possible To Follow Our Dreams?

Yes, it most definitely is very possible, and this is precisely what we should all be doing!

Do you have a dream of what you should be doing in life?

In your quiet alone moments do you see yourself living a radically different life to the one you currently lead?

In my case I am following my dream right now. Although it certainly hasn't always been this way!

My higher self for sure had a bit of a scream at me for quite a few years. Clear signs about what I should be doing with my life were presented to me. In increasingly simplistic and obvious ways, which I duly ignored. I am sure my higher-self must have thought I was either incredibly lazy or unbelievably stupid. Then eventually I decided I had better firstly write and then get out there and talk to people. Spread some love out into this World. Much to the relief of my higher self I am sure!

As we are becoming more aware of Energy or indeed it could be said, more spiritually aware, if our life is a little way off centre from our true potential, then it generally happens that there will be clear signs that what we are doing is not for us.

This can even often make it more or less impossible to continue upon our current pathway and absolutely force us to take a different direction. Sometimes we have to dismantle our current reality to forge a new one from out of the scattered remains of all we knew. It happens this way when we tend to ignore those inner urgings of our higher calling, triggering a necessary phoenix experience and we have to trust if this happens that, although the process can be confusing and traumatic, ultimately The Universe has our back and it is all happening for our own greater good.

It is possible to follow your dream. All I would say as a word of advice is to be sure you want it and that the dream is YOUR original thought about how you feel your ultimate reality should be.

It is all too easy to be influenced by the thoughts and wishes of those around us...

Over the course of our life, but especially in childhood as we learn about co-existing with our parents, siblings and then the bigger World, through school and socializing with our peers, we build up a series of unconscious automatic responses to what is going on around us.

These can be in terms of reacting in a way that is expected by others, even if this is not strictly how we really feel.

Moulding to the expectations of parents, teachers, friends...the result being that we are programming ourselves to react in certain ways. And this can be through the suppression of those emotions we truly feel about a situation, pushing our own feelings aside, in order to co-exist in harmony.

Another by product is to detach us from our centre. Who we are and what we need can get a little lost along the way.

I Digressed. Anyway, Back To Words

What we need to realise is that words have a great power of attraction.

Thoughts...then words.

And words spoken with great emotion have the absolute strongest power. What we say reflects how we feel about ourselves, shining out like a beacon to those who are aware of the way Energetic Reality works.

Highly judgemental or critical people are at some level unhappy with themselves, where they are in life and constantly project that onto others.

Angrily aggressive people are projecting outwardly their frustration with their own self-imposed feelings of limitation.

The professional cynic is not really feeling a lot of self-love.

At the other end of the scale, the truly centred, happy person, makes others feel better just for being in their presence. They send out warm pleasant energy into The Universe and the Law Of Attraction means this is what they get back in return.

If you observe the people you know and listen to what their general conversation contains you get a surprisingly good idea of where they are psychologically. How they feel about their life and themselves. What do they talk about and how do they look at others? It is more than possible by reading between the lines of how they express themselves to understand far more about them and maybe develop a little more compassion for their idiosyncrasies as a consequence.

When someone says something harsh or unpleasant to us all they are in fact they are doing is reflecting their own feelings about themselves onto us. It could be us or it could be the next person to cross their path and it is quite literally not personal.

If someone close to us is unkind and unpleasant, it is simply because we are conveniently close at hand and is still a reflection of how they feel about themselves and truly not about us.

If we ourselves are in the habit of putting down others or behaving in a way that is detrimental to feeling harmonious around people then we need to take a good look at why. Where does that reaction come from and what makes us behave in that way?

Has Your Money Got Good Or Bad Attitude?

Anyone can have financial freedom. It is not going to mean a lot if we are as miserable as the meanest miser though is it?

Money is there to be used and circulated around out into the world. Not for sitting on top of afraid to let it go. So anyone can have financial freedom.

"Is that so?" I can hear you asking. Yes! It definitely is!!!

It really is all about the attitude we have gotten into the habit of with money. That maybe it is in some way impossible to be financially rich and possess vast amounts of any kind of currency you can think of. I am here to say this is simply untrue and I am also willing to state that for that you will agree with me as you read on. That attitude is ALL when it comes to making it big financially.

Oh and to clarify here that I am not talking about winning the lottery, although I do get to many that would be kind of cool. I agree it would, but on the other hand I never do play the lottery...

What I am talking though about taking control yourself of your life by developing a different mindset. It would be easy to say the easiest way to keep money is by not spending any, but we have all got our commitments and needs to be met.

Do you ever think of yourself as being poor?

I guess we can all work out where that mindset is going to take us. We are going be poor. Poor is a state of mind and one that does not serve anyone in any way! If we are low on funds right now that is a temporary situation. And it's a situation that can quickly change for the better. Never ever ever ever think of yourself as poor! Ever!!!

The quickest way to turn around any financial situation is with some planning. If you are in debt, then you need to sit down and honestly work out a plan of how to clear the debt. One that is achievable in the shortest possible time, but also without leaving you with nothing left to live off! This can be organizing monthly amounts to pay, that you can afford to cover or cutting back on other spending until you are free of debt. Once you have cleared what you owe, then ensure that you never find yourself in the same situation. How? Do keep on reading! If you have got a credit card clearly never allow the balance to go over what you know you easily can pay back each month.

Something is going to have to crucially change and firstly we need to stop spending money unnecessarily.

I don't mean not enjoy your cash, obviously see to definite commitments firstly and then if there happens to be any left over by all means have that night-out or buy those shoes, but you still might want to leave a little over in your bank. So many people live beyond their means and on credit. Never has a happy ending. It has all got to be paid back some day...

Self-made entrepreneurs didn't go around splashing the cash on their way to success. Instead they spent their currency on things that will earn them more... money!

Investing in stuff that will make money is absolutely brilliant. I do it all the time and I can tell you the feeling is almost like magic, especially when it works!

I will tell you some of my own ongoing ways to material success later. For the moment though we have got to strike a happy balance between being cool to let money go or in other words spend when we need to and not wasting away our hard-earned cash. If we want to become successful then we obviously usually have to be prepared to spend some money to achieve this, so really think about where you are allocating your financial outgoings.

Only you can decide what really matters to you. Personally I love buying stuff to recycle or upcycle that I can sell for more then I paid for it - I find that amazing beyond what I ever thought possible.

Assets And Liabilities

Here is a fascinating question I usually ask during my talks which will generally provoke a passionate response from my audiences "What do you consider are the main material assets and liabilities in your life?"

Their answers on assets vary from cars, computers, homes, businesses, precious jewellery or any one of the other countless material items many of us value.

Typically their liabilities turn out to be bank or credit card loans to pay off, heavy mortgages or sometimes even their job!

Understandably there are many variations in fine detail within the answers my audiences offer as feedback, averagely though they do tend to narrow down to something along those similar themes.

Okay, time to again be a little candidly honest once more and risk courting controversy with these next statements All I ask is keep an open mind and I promise you will see where I am coming from here:

1.   Anything at all you are purchasing on any kind of a loan which will end up being worth less than you paid for it once the loan is complete and paid-up – this is a liability.

2.   Anything at all which adds material value to your life or somehow brings you closer to your ideal reality in any way, however indirectly or abstractly - this is an asset.

Stress is all too often directly caused by living beyond our means, paying too much for those things which bring us absolutely no closer to our goals and in fact end up being worth far less materially than we slogged away to purchase them for.

Been There, Done That, Learned The Lesson

When I first started to make a small profit for myself with my own first business (when I was done with working for others), out I went and treated myself to a beautiful silver Jaguar X-Type car on credit.

Quite effectively tying-up a few hundred of my working capital every single month to meet those re-payments. Money which might instead have been using to help grow my business through expanding my marketplace through buying advertising.

Quickly I came to look upon this car as entirely pointless. It sat right there in the car-park (depreciating more in value every week!) while I worked to pay for it. It precisely added nothing to my dreams, success mindset or for sure any sense of wellbeing. On the contrary I saw it as a large physical manifestation of a lesson learned and as soon as it was eventually paid for in full I promptly sold it the same day!

Being a car person, for many years before that Jaguar I would swap my car at regular intervals. Becoming a bit bored with what I had, I bought into the lifestyle adverts for new improved models and changed. Until the day when I sold on the Jaguar and I finally sat down and worked out exactly how much I had spent on cars over the previous twenty or so years. Let's just say I could have probably bought a small tropical island with the final total! And so, in horror at my own folly, instead I bought out of the consumerism...

At the time of writing I do still own a car, well okay two classic cars, one is twenty years old and the other is fort-three this year. They are kept serviced and repaired if necessary. They have never let me down and combined they originally cost me about 25% of the on-the-road price of that last new car. What's more they actually appreciate in value every single year!

Once we drive that new car out of the showroom and onto the road it has already shed a third of its value before we have even reached our own driveway to park.

New cars are nice to own (I should know!) for sure they make little financial sense, but I do agree they are seriously nice to own.

If our requirements dictate a good reliable modern car then far better buy a nearly new one that is under a year old. Choose wisely and they can still feel pretty much like new. All the big money in depreciation has already been shed by the first owner and what is even better we won't be making some car manufacturing corporation richer by ordering their latest product straight off the production line. And dramatically reducing our carbon footprint in the process. Talk about win/win!

Imagine if you and I were to sit down to have a chat over a decaf coffee to talk back about our spending over the last year.

- Just how many pieces of technology did we upgrade?

- Did the device it replace still work as intended when it was rendered obsolete by us?

- Is its replacement significantly better?

- How much over the course of an entire decade will these yearly tech-upgrading cost?

If this is anything like the total I spent on cars, I don't know about you, but I would rather allocate a little of my surplus cash to having experiences to enrich the lifestyle of my family like travelling to interesting places, rather than willingly giving it to a corporation who managed to persuade me to opt into their lifestyle dream (i.e. buy their stuff!)

Whenever we are tempted to change a still fully functioning piece of kit, if we remind ourselves that this was our one choice out of all the options available when we purchased it and so we must have rather good taste after all. And by keeping our perfectly working piece of kit we happily reduce our carbon footprint as a cool by-product of our choice.

Over To You

Ponder your own life, how many assets do you possess compared to liabilities?

At this point I know it won't be possible to change some things which you might well now be viewing as liabilities, rather than assets. Positively instead use this new-found perspective to inspire a long-term plan to turn around your life balance to possessing more assets than liabilities!

In the meantime, when we are making future financial commitments of any kind, honesty with ourselves pays long term dividends:

1. Will this commitment be a sound financial investment, in other words add value materially or in terms of helping to attain your goals in the fullness of time?

2.   If the answer is yes, great you are looking at an asset!

3.   If the answer is no, then you might want to seriously consider if this is something you really wish to buy-into or go ahead with.

Of course, once you have got unlimited funds available, absolutely indulge a little and treat yourself and your family to some of non-profit making luxuries they can enjoy!

We love to travel visiting inspiring places, having the freedom to visit art galleries of our choice around the world or experience places of natural beauty is food for our souls indeed. Money is made to be circulated around and enjoyed. And studying success will ensure this wonderful freedom happens without further delay...

By The Way

Your truly most valuable personal assets are never things, of course, they are right there in your skill-sets and imagination!

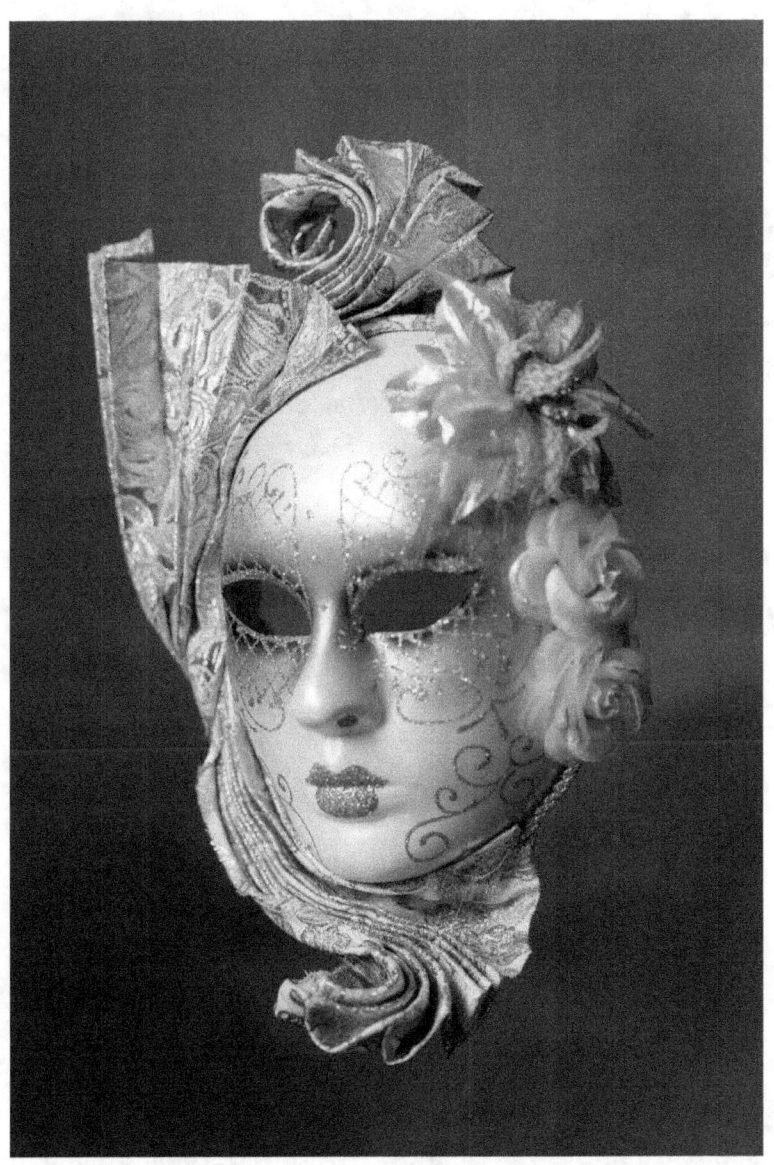

E-Commerce

As I have moved into full time writing and public speaking, most of my business interests these days are built around the internet in one way or another. Although my main work is basically helping others through my creative endeavours, as a serial entrepreneur I cannot resist still having one or two other businesses going at any given time.

E-shops and online bookstores reach markets a high street shop or even personal business website never could – well not without spending a few hundred thousand a year on advertising. I write books, record audiobooks and go out into the big wide world to deliver talks - I focus on what I love to do.

I appreciate how fortunate I am. I get to make a real difference in the experience others have in their lives. Yet I know in reality what I do is show others the latent potential they always possessed within themselves but didn't quite know how to apply in their day-to-day life.

Okay, so on to my most recent business venture. Let's talk about a famously well-known worldwide online auction site. Yikes! Dangerously close to straying into "scrimping book" territory here!

This is a little different though as I am not going to suggest selling all your unwanted garbage from your loft or garage to pay for your holidays. Instead I will share with you how I set up one of my own green eco-conscious businesses selling recycled stuff people seem to apparently endlessly wish to buy.

Perhaps I shouldn't be sharing this, after all I have done pretty well from it and if I go telling everyone they will all want a piece of the action! Oh what the heck, room for us all I guess...

Okay here is what sells ridiculously well on our famous auction site:

1. Children's DVDs.

2. 80's music cassettes.

3. 90's music CDs but only the rare ones individually or mixed job lots of popular titles.

4. Hardback factual books (cookbooks are best).

5. Children's clothes and shoes, but they must be a good label.

6. Branded toys.

And that is about it in my experience. I have people go along to thrift/charity shops/garage sales looking for all this stuff and then I re-sell it on the site. And it always sells!

I love recycling and getting involved in this online auction business was originally entirely motivated by my passion for the re-use and upcycling of other peoples discarded and unwanted stuff. I donate 10% of everything I make to charities, which feels to me like the right choice to make.

Well-Meaning Advice To Usually Ignore

Friends and family can for sure offer us much appreciated support within our endeavours by believing in what we are doing and morally supporting us to help us stay on track. Uncle Bob may be a wise and wonderful guy, but if he hasn't actually done what you want to do, chances are his advice will only be well-meaning opinions with no hard facts to back them up.

Far better we seek out those high-fliers within our field of endeavour and listen to what they might have to say. Those experts who have been there, done that and can offer real practical advice to guide us.

By the way, we are never obliged to HAVE to take their advice. The more feedback we can obtain though within any potential directions to take the easier it is to make decisions and ultimately the best way is still always opting to go with our intuition or that gut feeling.

In my own experience business advisors within banks and similar financial institutions may well be highly qualified, although crucially they have never usually physically run businesses or had any direct experience in dealing with the complexities of managing a team of employees. Do ensure to take the time to validate any advice you might get from business advisors at banks. Check it out with others who possess proven track-records with real experience of running business successes to call upon.

If you can't personally network with those top-of-the-tree movers and shakers in your career choice, instead absorb their autobiographies and watch online vids or vlogs if they have one. Step into their mindset to see what they might do faced with your choice.

The same goes for accountants, their financial advice may well be spot-on, but never take for granted that it is necessarily going to be right for you.

Be sure to take the time to ponder all practical options before making a commitment to any course of action which affects the long-term viability of your business venture and then go with your intuition in the end. And 99.9% of the time that will be the right choice...

Think Big!

It is a bit of a no -brainer that the way to make larger than life successes is to think big!

And yet so many potential success stories do limit what they can achieve with small-minded thinking or subconscious fear of real wealth. Okay, I sense some breaking down of barriers is going have to happen and see where it all goes, let's engender some trust in one another here.

Are you happy with the house you are currently living in or would you prefer somewhere that is a wee bit more shouting out YOU?

- Form a picture in your mind of your ideal house. What do you see?

- Might be a regency period detached house with some land or a villa overseas, could be a penthouse pad – whatever is your ideal house basically.

- Really think about this, go from room to room and see how it looks.

- Now double the size of your ideal house, add in whatever features you have always dreamed of.

- Could be a swimming pool, wall to wall clothes in your own dressing room, a gym, tennis courts or whatever else floats your boat.

- See how much more room you have got for all your stuff? Room to breathe and really chill.

- You are now thinking big!

And you can do the same with pretty much anything you see as your idea of success. Don't care if your goal or ambition is about how much you would like to earn each month or the kind of car you drive, it works just the same.

Okay salary next – however you are paid you can do this. Picture in your mind your usually salary, the actual figure. Now add another nought onto the end. Feels good doesn't it? Now add another nought onto the end. Dare to dream about having all the cash you could ever need and plenty left over to spread around however feels right to you.

Next on to your wheels. What do you drive right now? Happy with it? So go on what have you always wanted? A sports car, ecocar, limo or SUV or whatever else you are into – it is all about your personal taste here. Spend some time dreaming about what your perfect wheels would be. Think about sitting inside and looking out the windshield at the road. If you see one on a parking lot or the road imagine driving it. Okay, you might not be a position to go buy one right now, thing is though, by focusing on dreams and desires we all come that much closer to making them happen. It is about programming your mind to think in a wealth orientated way. Connecting mentally to the things we want makes them seem that much nearer and more possible. Oh, and you still might like to consider buying a nearly new car to reduce your carbon footprint rather than going along the brand-new route...

If you have your own business decide how big you want it to grow? Are you building it for yourself, your children's future or have you got an exit strategy in mind to sell the business on at some point?

Push back the boundaries of what you can achieve with your business. If you are building it to sell on at some point you are going to need to come up with a plan to make this real such as a timescale; and everything you do can then lead to making it happen. If you are growing it for yourself or your children, step back from time to time and see if there any ways you can get into new marketplaces and achieve new kinds of success.

In Other Words THINK BIG!

I have actually heard friends say they would like to have more money, but not too much. Perhaps a few hundred thousand, but not something like millions, that would be way too stressful!

Oh really?! How exactly?

All they want to do is pay off their mortgage, send their children through Uni, get a newer car and maybe catch a few good vacations. These friends are limiting themselves completely and totally. Setting low targets about what they want to achieve. And they could do so much more…

Becoming financially successful can open so many doors. It is also going lead to a complete lifestyle change. We do have to be prepared for the fact that having greater wealth does bring more responsibility, for sure.

You are going to need to employ a good accountant to reduce your taxable funds and you will need to decide what you are going do with your success; invest in property, businesses, buy shares etc,. This is what those guys are scared of, they don't want this kind of pressure and so they limit themselves.

The tricks to building wealth are learned as you go along. The advice of strategic accountants and PA's can always be listened to, but it is always your gut instinct you would be wisest to go with in the end.

Nowadays it is commonly recognised the company we keep creates a tremendous impact on exactly how we view the world. We end up coming to the same level as those main friends we hang-out with the most, socially, emotionally and economically. In a real sense our crowd can help or hinder us, it all depends.

How often have those who achieved overnight success found their immediate circle of influence change accordingly. This new-found success of theirs being so far removed from many old acquaintances comfort zones they cannot remain friends, no common ground existing anymore. We do need to be prepared for this possibility happening.

See It Clearly

Can you imagine yourself living that ideal life? Dreams you have held onto for so many years, finally acted upon and coming to be your reality? The utopia you always secretly thought was possible excitingly becoming your everyday direct experience.

It doesn't matter if rather like a game of snakes and ladders getting there might not always take the most direct route. It is the pictures in your own minds eye of where you will eventually be and the utter belief in the reality of your life once you are there which ensures your dreams can go all the way and you will stay on track, whatever happens.

We never need to see every step beforehand which will lead us there, planning it all out stops those leftfield opportunities from being grabbed.

Look Like A Million Dollars

Cliché alert!

"Dressing for Success" makes you feel more successful.

It really seriously does!

Don't you feel better when you are wearing your best stuff and know you are looking good?

If the answer to that is no or you don't have any "best" clothes then I can see we are going to need to have a little talk before we move on.

If you look like you are successful then you soon notice that you will start being treated differently. People will be more courteous and definitely more interested in what you have to say. This has to be good for anyone who is wealth seeking, think about it...

If other people believe that you are successful and/or wealthy then they are going to be constantly reflecting that image back onto you and so if they are buying into it then you can soon make it happen for real.

You need to decide which style of dressing and fashion makes you personally feel like a winner. Could be a favourite designer label, a smart business suit, sportswear; or even copying as an example anyone who is globally successful in whatever field you work in (but only if you like their style and will feel comfortable wearing it).

Whatever Works For You And You Associate With Success

If your current financial reality makes it impossible to wear Prada, doesn't matter one little bit. Pay a visit to one of the better kinds of thrift/charity shops or hit the internet auction sites, the classy ones. They will always happily sell you some amazing bargains of virtually unworn top-end designer labels at a fraction of the new price. Shop around on a budget and you will find yourself putting super-models to shame with the labels you are wearing. And no need to tell anyone where you got all of your kick-ass outfits from, just enjoy the feeling.

When I started out in business I got myself a few perfect Yves Saint Laurent shirts from an online auction site, for something like 15% of the high street price and you can imagine how they made me feel incredibly successful when I was out and about making deals...

Okay, to be honest these shirts were positively psychedelic so don't necessarily wear ones like these! Personally, they worked well for me but could be considered a little far-out for some tastes; then again I do tend to dress a little like a member of a 1960's psychedelic rock band who time travelled into the modern day! Not for nothing have I been labelled by the press the Hippie Holistic Lifestyle Coach.

Find something true to you and then wear it brilliantly!

If you have got to wear overalls or a uniform for work you can still make a difference. Buy some killer designer underwear or some top-end perfume/cologne; you are still going feel different than before and more successful.

Shoes also make a difference; how the heck can you feel like a winner if they are all scuffed or down at heel?

Invest some cash in your look; it will pay you back many times over and you can thank yourself later!

Find Something You Will Love To Do

Too many people who could be great achievers go through life doing basically nothing. No direction or inspiration ever shakes them out of their deadly boring routine.

What I am going give you are a few clues to yourself on how to become your very own success story by following your gut instinct or intuition.

I believe that we all possess this kind of inbuilt radar. Deep down we ALWAYS know if something is right or wrong for us. The trouble is a lot of us have become rather good at ignoring our intuition and only going with what logically seems the right choice...

Time for a full stop, line drawn under and goodbye to all that!

If more people went with their gut feeling instead of logic there would be many happier more fulfilled people out there.

Self-made millionaires, and I don't care how cautious they might apparently seem, will still follow their intuition. And if something just doesn't feel right they won't touch the deal no matter what.

So What Would You Like To Spend Your Days Actively Doing?

We have all got something we can excel at, something we have maybe dreamt of doing and yet never allowed ourselves to ponder it could actually happen for real.

It is incredibly important to earn your living doing something that you feel passionate about and you love. You are going to need a notepad and pen (not an electronic notepad please, a real pen and paper works better for this).

Write down any particular talents you feel you may have. Don't be shy here, you could be a great organizer, math may be your thing, perhaps you are a fabulous communicator or able to see the bigger picture. Be honest and write any talents you feel you possess down on your pad in a list.

Next look at your list, and I am assuming you have written a few things down by now and if you haven't managed to yet you are going want to give it some more thought!

I will give you a moment or two longer...come back when you have something written down...right...

Now, looking at your list have a think about what kind of careers can let you use your natural talents and write them alongside.

After all, if you think about it, how cool would it be to be working in some career you are awesome at doing? Plus, if this is using your natural abilities you are halfway there to being successful before you even start and you will consistently enjoy what you do within your career.

So, you have now got a list of your talents and how they can be used. All you have need do now is choose something from the list and you possess that most valuable of assets…A GOAL IN LIFE!

Okay, so what if this is something you need to get qualifications for? Not got time to study full-time. Then take an e-course or part-time study. Got to be worth it to get where you want to be, yes?

Or maybe you don't need any qualifications, only your own talents and a good dose of enthusiasm. What next?

It is no use having a brilliant plan for business, but you are clueless how to go about getting it all started. Speak to people who do know and they will help you.

Join business networking forums or real-life business clubs. Ask for advice and 99.9% of times more experienced businesspeople will help you. You would be surprised how helpful networking can be, especially if it is obvious to others you are serious about your plans.

It can cost virtually nothing to gain shed loads of wisdom from more experienced businesspeople, who will usually be happy to pass on their wisdoms to someone just starting out. Your local Chamber of Commerce usually offers free advice as well. As do business advisors at banks, but as we discussed earlier, do bear in mind those guys might never have actually run a business, only worked in banking. Don't be afraid to ask for advice but remember always follow that gut feeling in the end.

Some Business Common Sense

If a little of my own story can help anyone else I am happy to care and share. I will simply tell you what has worked for me and what I have learned about hiring people...

Hiring People First

Qualifications are wonderful and can certainly look impressive. Guess how many self-made millionaires studied business at Uni? Hardly any at all that I know of. Instead they got out there into the real world and learned for themselves. I am not being down on education here; obviously, it is crucially important for specialist subjects like accountancy, healthcare or law.

Yet I have had many Uni graduates come along to see me armed with their business studies or psychology degrees and they fail to impress me just because they are packing a big degree.

I am far more interested in enthusiasm and how well they will integrate into the team. Enthusiasm is crucially important to achieve anything. I don't care if a candidate has first class honours degrees in management from a top Uni, if they shake hands like a wet rag and can barely raise a smile on their face when I talk with them they are not going find their way into employment so easily. Not with me anyway!

Failing Our Way To Success

By the way, the times I have fallen on my face with a business is when I have sort of known at some level it isn't working but refused to accept this reality and stubbornly carried on trying to force it to succeed. Sometimes you have got to know when to quit. Turn away from that particular dream and close the chapter in the most mutually beneficial way.

Ethics

It goes without saying that screwing people over in business is never a good idea. The business world is not as big many people think (even at a global level) so if someone goes around intentionally doing bad deals, sooner or later it will for sure turn around and bite them!

Most of my business interests these days are built around the internet in one way or another. It is possible to sell to billions of potential customers around the world now and I passionately love selling. Online auction sites reach markets a high street shop or even personal business website never could – well not without spending a few hundred thousand a year on advertising. I like music, toys and books, so this is what I mainly sell.

I have got other business interest as well, but it is so cool making profits you can easily see and I love providing excellent customer service. Stick to promises you make and you are doing things pretty much the right way.

Make A Timescale And Set Targets

Set yourself targets, make a list to tick them off one by one as you achieve them. A timescale makes your plans real, gives you something to aim for and you are going to love that high when you have done it!

It is way too easy to drift along dreaming, make a realistic timescale written down and get started now.

The other point is you have need to have at least some idea what you are setting out to achieve. I know it as kind of difficult to predict what exactly is going to happen, especially with no framework of experience to fall back on.

What you do need to decide though is to be clear what you personally want to happen say one month down the line, three months, six months and so on.

This doesn't necessarily have to be rigidly stuck to. Your targets may well be revised as you learn more about your business. Whatever targets you do set though need to be high, but definitely achievable!

Always set targets, for the business, yourself, and your employees if you have any. That way everyone knows what is expected of them. And when targets are reached and another milestone passed, the feeling of elation is worth all the hours put in and the sacrifices.

If your timescale and targets seem to be falling behind a bit, you will need to look at and analyse why this is happening and correct it, so you can then carry on with your progress.

Stay Focused And You Will Get There!

If you have taken on board what you have read so far I am trusting that you now possess a clearer picture in your mind on where you want your life to go.

Yet it can be so easy to lose track and the sight of dreams. Everyday distractions come along and suddenly boring old life patterns are fallen back into and progress stops dead.

Okay, you are going need some prompting reminders focussed on why you are doing what you what you do. They reasons why you want more from life!

Find a home screen on your pc, mac and phone which inspires you. Could be a quote or picture that brings to life something to do with your goals. Like a cool house or relating to the lifestyle you want. Whatever makes you personally feel good about what you are aiming for.

Leave post it notes on your mirrors, fridge door, car dashboard - basically anywhere you will see them a lot. Keep prompting yourself to think in a different way and for sure it is going to happen sooner or later!

Thinking big needs to become a second nature type of thing all the time. Spotting opportunities and being ready to act upon them.

Physically connect to all the trappings of success you are making happen. Read about the type of houses you want to own – or whatever else you desire to have in your life.

You are aligning your thoughts and subconscious mind to make all these things seem very real and possible.

If you want to travel, then read travel books and look at travelogue websites. If you can't yet afford the trip you want, instead go and buy the suitcase or backpack instead! You are then preparing yourself for when you can then...

If you want at Bentley, buy an official Bentley keyring. Take a test-drive then you know what the experience feels like first-hand.

Why not surround yourself with pictures of all the things you are sure to have really soon? Make them part of your décor.

Whatever they are such as mansions, big yachts, private jets or more designer labels than you could ever wear. Whatever motivates you personally. Every time one of the pictures catches your eye imagine you are connected to leading that life not shortly...but now! And then believe it can actually happen because you are taking the action to make it your life!

What Matters Most? The Greener Option...

I guess like most reasonably sane people I believe it is right and correct to preserve this precious planet upon which we rely to live. In this chapter we will go through a few examples of how to turn away from mass consumerism and happily reduce our carbon footprint in the process.

I am certainly not perfect; I do drive and also travel a fair amount as part of my vocation and for pleasure. And yet, even taking a few steps to living within a greener consciousness will for sure make a difference within the bigger picture.

We can only do our best within our current lifestyle choices...and if when we achieve this kind of balance and harmony, then we naturally find ourselves automatically motivated to do more.

Remaining Authentically True To Ourselves

Control how anyone emotionally responds, and you control the person.

Our own moral framework is governed by our emotional responses to different experiences and situations. Naturally, these evolve through time, along with our maturity and experience. What served us well in terms of reactions at eighteen is hardly likely to work quite the same for us at forty or fifty.

What is normally consistent regardless of age though is through our interaction with the outside world, how these personal built-in responses makes us feel, which determines our own personal code of ethics. As we go through life we are bombarded with often very subtle messages telling us what to buy, what to believe, where to go on holiday, how good life could be if we bought whatever is being sold, and what is even considered "normal"!

These gentle persuaders don't come only from typical methods like adverts, they are usually far wider reaching than that. Mass media and popular culture are amongst some of the ways of controlling our lifestyle habits, encouraging us to go buy and creating the need within people for ever more material goods.

Now before you all throw this book down or delete it in horror at the suggestion that you might not benefit that latest smart-phone you just bought or your favourite magazine might be primarily selling you stuff, I want to ask you to humour me here and read on until the end. As well as reducing our carbon footprint we might even save you some of your hard-earned cash along the way...

Are You IN?

This beautiful planet is after all our only physical home, then has to be a no-brainer that it makes sense to cherish and love it. A small carbon footprint can only be good.

Sadly, not all of our fellow residents of Gaia share this opinion. They have an altogether different range of motivations.

Public companies and corporations employ whole teams of marketing experts whose job description is to find as many different ways as possible to encourage us to spend with them.

They achieve this by creating a need.

If we see our favourite actor or singer wearing a brand of clothing chances are we will subconsciously judge it to be cool. Possibly even looking to purchase for ourselves whatever we saw next time we go clothes shopping. The difference here is that Jay Z and his friends will be paid mega-bucks to wear that stuff and we have to instead lay out mega-bucks to wear it as well!

Mobile phones are blanket marketed. If we have a perfectly functioning phone that we are basically happy with this is not going to make phone manufacturers more profitable. So they come up with evolutions and improvements; the idea being to make us feel like our model is now obsolete and just a little bit sad to still be using. Far better we go throw it in the trash right now and get their new cool upgraded phone instead. They are allegedly some major players in the smartphone industry who intentionally downgrade the speed and capability of their phones out there still being used after a little while; making us feel we really must upgrade as our current phone is now so slow.

Okay, I will admit for a little while I bought into this phone upgrade scam. Buying for myself a smart-phone which I won't name and shame. This looked awesome and worked simply fine until I actually wanted to make a call from my own home. I genuinely found I needed to stand on my bed to get any kind of signal!

Returning to the shop a few weeks later to ask for an explanation from the staff, to be told by the salesperson "Better to upgrade to the newer version of that phone. That old model has been replaced by this one with one with more apps and it's available in all these cool new colours". All I wanted was a phone to principally receive and make calls on, maybe text a bit and also check my emails.

I then bought out of the phone rat race and got myself the cheapest phone I could find and guess what? I can make calls on it, send texts as well and go online! Keeping our low tariff phone for years doesn't make any profit for phone companies - cool!

Some new version on any gadget is always being introduced with the intention of making us feel like our existing model is something our stone-age ancestors would have been happy using.

If what we already have works perfectly well why on earth should we trash it and upgrade? Just makes corporations richer in the process and leaves us with something doing exactly the same job as the old version we binned, just in some alleged cool new colour or with some little extra bling? And it is going to look so last year in six months' time anyway and then it all begins again...

Welcoming Home

The same rules apply to home furnishings and by this, I mean everything we usually buy for the home including sofas, new kitchens, bathrooms, and the whole range of soft furnishings. Our grandparents when they were starting out life together would have gradually bought all these things, expecting them to last a lifetime and invariably they would.

Instead now we have the home "make-over experience" that many of us on average undertake every five years give or take.

As décor becomes "unfashionable", bathrooms and kitchens get ripped out to be taken along to the local landfill site, together with sofas and all the other now obsolete things that five years ago seemed so chic. And we spend plenty of cash replacing it all with the latest trends; probably to then do it all again in another five years' time. And the manufacturers are happy.

How about fitting out our homes with décor that ultimately reflects only our own taste and style?

Totally ignore and bypass the latest trends...

We both know that is all they will be...trends. Always have been, always will be.

Go instead with surrounding ourselves with things we will love to live with every day. By buying right out of fashion, our homes are never going to date or look like the discarded set from a sit-com tv show from ten years ago; instead they will have a timeless kind of appeal.

The only time it will be necessary to upgrade is when something actually gets worn out and genuinely needs to be replaced (or if we are at long last thoroughly sick of the sight of the item and we can then donate it to a charity for them to sell on!)

Fashionably Bohemian

Fashion next. I have a fashion superhero, my sister-in-law. She decides what she wants to wear and goes along to her usual ethical clothes store. Seeing what she came for, which is usually up there at the top end of prices, she then travels home. And goes online. She looks around to see if it is available anywhere else for less than the store price. If it isn't, she waits. Every time she goes into the city she revisits the store, to check the price. Once it is time for the winter sale, she will find the store is selling off end of season stock and she finally buys what she wanted for often just 20% of the considerable original price.

I am not suggesting everyone could be patient enough to do that or indeed that you need to "shop around to get a bargain" as that is just patronizing you.

Maybe you could wait a week or so though, just to have a looksee if the price does drop at all. Can't do any harm to give it a go. I have started doing like my sister-in-law, as much as my own patience will allow.

Although as an auction-site entrepreneur myself I do most of my shopping on-line, the same rule applies here though. And I have grabbed some absolute bargains over the years.

With an eye to my carbon footprint, I tend to only buy new clothes which I would be happy to still be wearing in five years. If something fits this category then I cheerfully go ahead and buy it. If not, then it won't generally find its way into my wardrobe.

Cars Again

For a start, how about making fuelling combustion engine cars greener? The technology already exists to move away from burning fossil fuels. Diesel engines will run on vegetable oil-based biofuel.

I found it would be necessary to take undertake a one-hundred-mile round trip if I opted to fuel my own diesel-powered car with biofuel. Although there is now a cut-off date for combustions engines being phased out, all those existing cars are not going to suddenly vanish into thin air! How about making biodiesel, made from vegetable oil, more widely available and then we can all collectively reduce our carbon footprint?

And while we are on the subject, why are solely electrically powered cars so ridiculously over-priced? I am not talking about hybrids here; I mean purely electric cars.

Can it really cost that much to manufacture them? They are constructed largely from polymers and mass-produced moulded plastic after all, what can be in them that makes them so expensive? The batteries? Really, can they genuinely cost all those tens of thousands of any currency we might choose to manufacture them?

With the current plug-in to charge electric cars, how can we be sure charging them is genuinely reducing our carbon footprint? Not everyone has access to solar panels on their houses and plugging them into the national grid across the country is risky at best for the greener option.

Doesn't it rather defeat the object of going electric if these zero-emission vehicles cause even greater indirect pollution than their combustion engine ancestors by relying upon power stations to charge them?

The technology exists to produce other types of zero-emission cars such as hydrogen-cell and hybrid hydrogen/electric, perhaps this might be the way to go instead? These cars only produce water as emissions. Investment in their development will ensure easier and more cost-effective, clean production of the necessary technology to fuel them. Rather than relying on the single choice for the future being solely plug-ins with their limited range and Co2 producing reliance on power stations.

It will be interesting to see where green-vehicle development goes over the next ten to twenty years and the direction investment takes.

Magazines

I spent my time working on both trade and consumer magazines, at one point owning my own publishing house.

Magazines survive from advertising. The cover price is not how the publisher makes their profit, which only usually covers the distribution costs. Advertising is what pays for the printing and how the staff's wages are covered. Clearly the editor has a duty of care to the advertisers to promote their products or services; if they are kept happy they will then continue to support the magazine, and everyone can stay in employment.

Companies send freebies to magazine journalists, gifts of all kinds, with the intention to subsequently receive reviews and editorial coverage. During my career I witnessed arriving at the office amongst many other things - full crates of fine wine and beer, cosmetics of every possible kind, food hampers often containing chocolate, vitamins, aloe-vera juice, fashion items of every conceivable type and rather bizarrely even coconut milk; all with the intention of buying a mention and some column space in the magazine. This would invariably work.

I am not suggesting for one moment this is always necessarily a terrible thing. After all how are we supposed to know about any new products that are being launched unless they get some kind of publicity?

The other point to consider here is if we enjoy our favourite magazines, does it really matter if some of the articles are in effect advertorials for various companies, if they are still essentially entertaining us?

Independent magazines will usually possess a degree of integrity and at least some of the original personal who passionately started the publication will be there involved in putting it together. The core values remain intact and they are true to the original vision of why they chose to start the magazine in the first place. Sure there will be commercial realities to face, but the balance is generally about right.

At the other end of the scale, most successful big glossy magazines are owned by gigantic media corporations. Your favourite read will just be one of many titles within their portfolio, which might also typically include commercial radio stations and tv/film businesses; and they will all need to show a good profit or be dropped.

As such the stressed staff will be employed to achieve profit and the result is they may not always have exactly the best interests of their readership at heart. To stay in employment, they are required to play the corporate game, and this will involve ensuring the big sponsors of the magazines, the ones who block-book advertising across all of the group's media (such as car manufacturers or phone companies) are continually passively promoted via their editorials. The staff will be employed to achieve profit above all else. Or to put it another way, they probably already sold their soul and grandmother a long time ago along with their integrity!

The 21st century does see many paper-only magazines struggling to survive, the harsh commercial reality of competition from free e-zines and the personal blogs of those we used to read about in magazines, rendering it increasingly challenging to exist.

I am a columnist, writing each year for over thirty magazines across the world; their wise shift to also providing downloadable e-editions of their magazines ensures they remain relevant and competitive.

Thriving!

Let's take a moment to think about those unfortunate souls whose only contact with others is through some secondary electronic device like a laptop or their smartphone.

The guy who consider 'likes' to actually mean something. Our guy has loads of online friends through social media although he has never actually met any of them or has any really genuine friends in the real world.

Surrounded By Concrete And Steel

Surviving as he does (can it accurately be described as living?) in a world dominated by electronic equipment, surrounded by bricks and concrete. Our guy spends his entire leisure time on his device/smartphone or playing computer games, only encountering vegetables and fruit when visiting the huge steel and glass supermarkets; the countryside is that green blur he momentarily views through the side windows of buses or seen flashing-by from the seat of a train.

A self-created reality existing in a complete and total sensory deprivation world. Never experiencing the pleasure of real conversations with fellow humans or feeling the joy of simply being alive!

Everything in our guy's immediate surroundings is unnatural and synthetically mass produced. All his direct experiences obviously also then become manufactured in some way.

Existing in this artificially created outside-of-reality bubble makes our guy extremely receptive to auto-suggestion. With no natural grounding point to lock onto to act as an anchor he becomes literally a cog in part of the bigger machine. An automated breathing consumer unit...

Our Natures

Why are we here on this planet at this moment?

What might be yours or indeed my mission in this life?

Surely it cannot be to simply work, opting out of any direct experience, eventually to then die leaving behind hardly any contribution to the betterment of the world?

No real trace of having been here other than our bloodline continuing...

Don't you feel we all deserve better?

I know I do and trust you feel the same way!

Yes, of course you and I deserve to live life to the full and enjoy every day whatever twists and turns it might take. To be true to our own ethics and morals. Have some fun, which might well cost absolutely nothing in hard cash, but is purely priceless.

Now that is living!

Think of walking in a forest after a fresh shower of rain, those heady scents and the sounds of birdsong high above in the trees.

Sitting by a seashore as waves loudly crash in on the beach or perhaps soothingly lap gently onto the shore.

The beauty of visually taking in a meadow full of a kaleidoscope of wildflowers.

The drama of a wild thunder-storm.

Looking up as an eagle majestically soars against a stunning sunset.

To be out on a crisp winters evening, the sky purest black and a million stars twinkling like diamonds.

Or a scorching hot summer's day, feeling the sun warming on our backs and experiencing true contentment.

This is real life!

This is directly appreciating freely given beauty, the beauty of nature, of our own natures and it is all waiting right there as it always has been. Waiting for you and I to feel it through all of our senses, with every breath down into every atom of our very being!

So, what would you rather enjoy?

Any one of these amazing natural experiences or spending time, like our guy does, on a device?

Why not go take a walk instead?

The countryside might be too far away, this need not be an issue. Public parks were created for us to use. Observe nature in all her beauty and wonder.

I believe if we all did this at least a couple of times a week, preferably more, but at least a couple of times, then we would feel fundamentally better within ourselves and naturally begin to focus more on our own wellbeing.

The more of us out there living fulfilled lives focussed on those things which truly matter, the happier the collective group mind becomes.

Our individual happiness can never be bought through acquiring things; it is about you and I making the personal choice to live on our own terms every single day and right there is our real key to lasting happiness!

Afterword

If you are now questioning yourself and your choices so far in your life, then looking around to see how you might more authentically live and go on to make your mark on life, then this book has done its job.

I choose not to be on social media, however, if you would like to know more or get in touch you can visit my official.

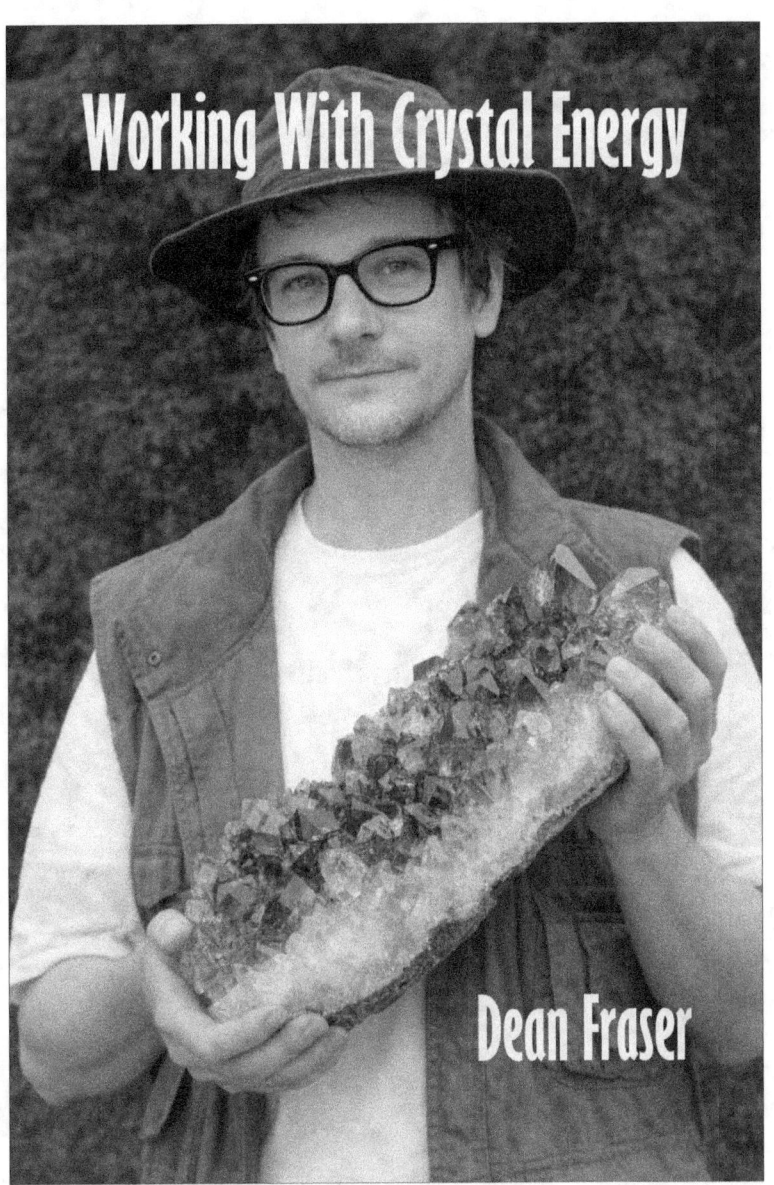

Working With Crystal Energy

Dean Fraser

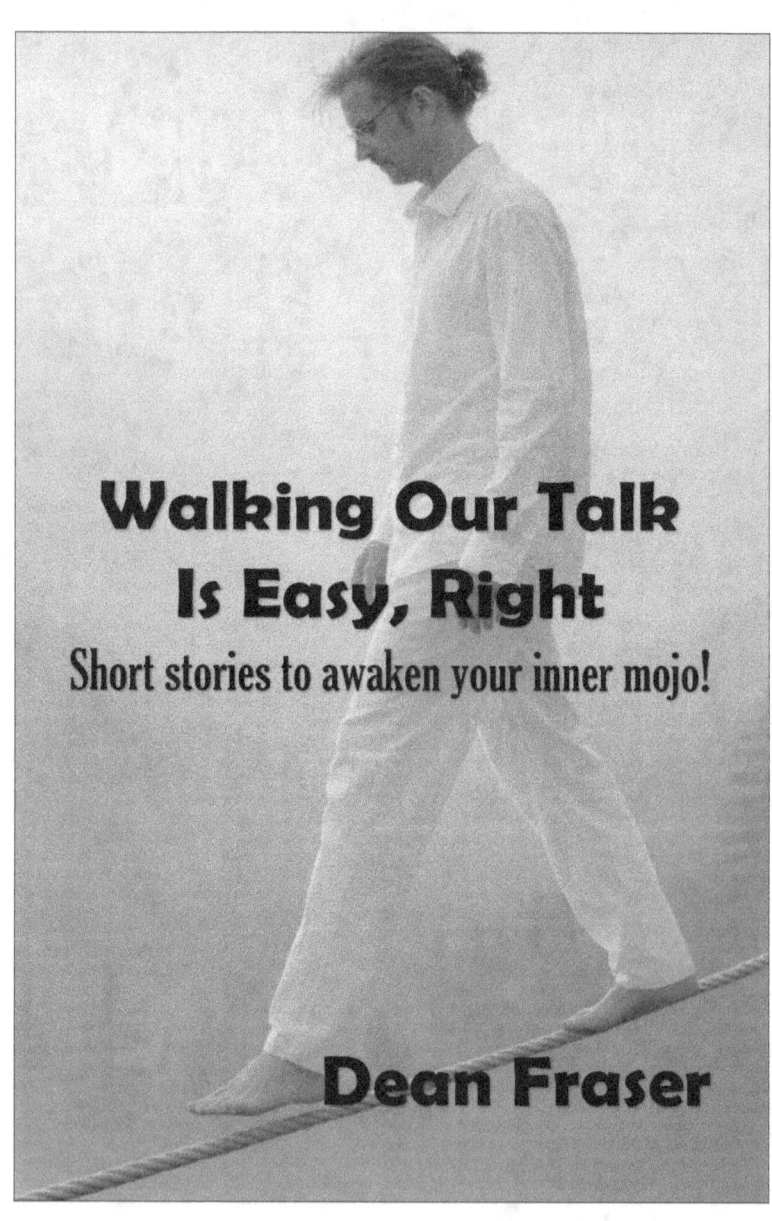

Walking Our Talk
Is Easy, Right

Short stories to awaken your inner mojo!

Dean Fraser

www.ingramcontent.com/pod-product-compliance
Lightning Source LLC
Chambersburg PA
CBHW071210280526
45787CB00002B/630